Introduction to Meditation
- Weight Management Series

Volume 4

Excerpt from Adopting a healthy lifestyle (1-884711-34-0)

Introduction to Meditation
- Weight Management Series

C.T. Pam

Copyright © 2013 by C. T. Pam

Published and printed in the United States by Innovative Publishers, Inc., Boston, Massachusetts.

Library of Congress Control Number: 2012922833

1-884711-76-6 978-1-884711-76-3 Paperback

Also available in the following formats

1-884711-77-4 978-1-884711-77-0 Kindle
1-884711-78-2 978-1-884711-78-7 Hardback
1-884711-79-0 978-1-884711-79-4 AudioBook
1-884711-80-4 978-1-884711-80-0 iBook
1-884711-81-2 978-1-884711-81-7 Nook

Printed in the United States of America

10 9 8 7 6 5 4 3 2 1   13 14 15 16

First edition, February 2013

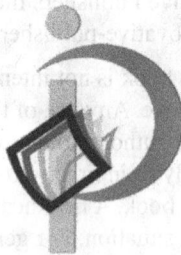

Innovative Publishers

Table of contents

Table of contents

Introduction to Weight Management

With the rapid rate at which obesity has spread over the last couple of decades, the importance of weight management programs has also grown as a consequence. Weight management program refers to all those activities that help an individual to either gain weight, lose weight or even to maintain it at the current level. In any of these goals, a weight management program targets increasing or maintaining the amount of lean muscle mass while decreasing the body fat percentage. Any other way of losing or gaining weight will be unhealthy in one aspect or another and may compromise health in the short term, but definitely in the long run.

Body Composition

Our body comprises of different components, namely fat, lean muscle, water, bones, organs etc. Each of them contributes to the total body weight. For each and every individual each of these constituent elements is present in different proportions. The ratio in which this distribution is present in any individual is called body composition. In the context of weight management, the division is done into two categories – fat mass and fat free mass. A healthy body composition is one in which the fat mass is low and fat free mass is higher. Through different weight management programs it is attempted to alter body composition in a manner that it boosts good health.

There are many techniques and methods to determine body composition. With technological advancements newer and more accurate equipments are available for performing body composition analysis. Traditional techniques such as skin fold measurements are easy to implement but have limited accuracy. Newer technologies such as ultrasound and bioelectric impedance analysis help in doing body composition analysis using simple and portable machines that give extremely accurate results as well. These different methods determine not only the amount of fat and lean muscle tissue but also provide a segmental analysis so that appropriate intervention strategies can be planned as part of the weight management program.

Doing body composition analysis on a regular basis should be included as part of any weight management strategy since it will help in monitoring the alterations taking place in the body as a result of the program. Since the body is undergoing change on a regular basis it is imperative that the program should also change accordingly. A program that was designed for the individual who weighed say 240 pounds will need to be changed when the person loses weight and weighs 200 pounds now. Body composition analysis also provides information on whether the weight loss is happening in a healthy manner or not. In case the weight loss happens at the expense of lean muscle or water then changes need to be done in the program so that these components can be restored to normal levels and fat loss targeted by introducing appropriate changes. A number of new age weight loss methods as well as gadgets are able to provide good results in terms of weight loss but they do it at the expense of good health. Doing a simple body composition analysis will reveal the true nature of these unhealthy methods and systems. Most new technologies also provide information on metabolic rate which is directly correlated the amount of lean mass in the body. Greater the lean mass higher will be the energy that is required by the body to maintain it. The measurement of metabolic rate helps in designing the exercise program as well as the calorie intake required as part of the diet & nutrition plan. Since the needs and requirement of each and every individual are different, the weight management strategy has to be necessarily different as well. Body composition analysis is the first step in designing a weight management program and should thereafter be done on a regular basis.

Problems with adverse body composition

A body composition analysis that reveals high fat percentage in comparison to lean muscle mass percentage points to obesity. Obesity is a modern day lifestyle disease that is essentially a silent killer. It indirectly leads to other physical as well as mental disorders, ailments and diseases that later on deplete the quality of life of the individual and in certain cases may even lead to death. The most common ailments that accompany obesity include type-2 diabetes, hypertension, cardiovascular & coronary artery disease, metabolic syndrome polycystic ovary syndrome and Dyslipidemia. Obesity also leads to gastrointestinal issues such as Cholelithiasis, GERD or Gastroesophageal Reflex Disease, Fatty Liver Disease, Colon Cancer and Hernia; genitourinary problems include erectile dysfunction, renal failure, incontinence and hypogonadism; Respiratory problems include sleep apnea, Hypoventilation syndrome and dyspnea. Apart from these physical ailments obesity also leads to psychological problems that arise from a diminished self confidence and if left unchecked may even lead to chronic depression.

Causes of Obesity

Obesity is caused by an energy intake in the form of diet that is not balanced by equivalent amount of physical activity. The basic law of conservation of energy cannot be violated at any cost and hence, energy excess will lead to weight gain while energy deficit will lead to weight loss. Energy input into the body is through the food that we eat. Energy output is the sum of a number of parameters that include – energy expended through physical exercise, energy spent in activities performed in daily life, basal metabolic rate or the energy required by the body to perform essential body functions such as respiration and digestion; in addition there are a few other parameters such as *thermic effect of food* and *adaptive thermogenesis* that add onto energy output but only in relatively small amounts. It is when the energy input becomes greater than energy output that the body starts storing this excess energy in the form of body fat. Some amount of fat is essential for efficient body functioning but when the fat percentage goes above certain levels it leads to obesity and consequently a host of other disorders and diseases.

This energy imbalance is the objective reason behind obesity but it is important to understand the underlying reasons why this imbalance is created. Imbalanced diet and sedentary lifestyle are the primary causes which get accentuated as a result of numerous personal, social, cultural and familial issues. Genetics and medical conditions also contribute towards increasing the fat mass in an individual. While most parameters seem to be alterable, some of these parameters may not seem to be in control of the individual and a situation of helplessness may be experienced. However, there are ways and means to counter any of these issues that gradually lead to weight loss in a healthy manner.

Genetic factors and Body Type

As mentioned above certain parameters that influence body composition cannot be modified. Genetic predisposition is one such parameter. Genetics define the body type of an individual which then affects the way in which the body reacts to a certain lifestyle and also to any alteration that is forced on this lifestyle. There are different classification techniques for differentiating between different body types.

1. The ancient Indian science of *Ayurveda* uses a classification method based on energy patterns or types. It is believed as per *Ayurveda* that the universe comprises of five basic elements – space, air, water, fire and earth. A combination of these basic elements is responsible for defining the human physiology. The basis of classification therefore is on the basis of energy patterns or *doshas* which comprise of one or more of these elements. The three *doshas* – *vata, pitta* and *kapha* define the person's physiology and all *Ayurvedic* treatments start from the identification of the *dosha* and identifying the imbalance in the *dosha* pattern. Once this is done remedial solution can be prescribed the aim of which is to restore the balance in the elements.

2. The second classification technique is based on the metabolic type. Under this classification technique the basis of differentiation between body types is the dominating gland in the endocrine system. It is believed that the biochemical reactions happening in the body of the individual are influenced and controlled by the dominating gland. This dominance of one particular gland over the others is built into the genetic structure and has a significant impact on the metabolic processes in the body. These metabolic processes take up raw materials such as carbohydrates, fats, proteins in different proportions and occur in the presence of catalysts that are available through micronutrients such as minerals and vitamins. The difference in proportions of raw material

utilized is due to the functioning differences between these glands of the endocrine system. The classification is done into 4 main categories – adrenal (controls reaction to environmental stresses and dangers), gonad (controls reproduction and growth), thyroid (controls metabolism) and pituitary (control the secretion of all glands) depending upon the dominating gland. Different diets and exercise routines are recommended for different body types.

3. The third classification technique and most commonly used in the context of weight management programs is on the basis of Somatotype. The system is based on identifying the association between psychological behavior patterns or temperament with the body structure of the individual. Under this system it is believed that the characteristic behavioral patterns as exhibited by an individual are typical of his or her own body type to a significantly large extent. The body type as in other classification systems is genetically predetermined. People having a similar body type are expected to show similar behavioral traits under this system. The system of classification is on the basis of the 3 elements or Somatotypes that are named after cell groups known as *germinal epithelium* formed during the growth of the embryo in the womb. The three Somatotypes are named after the three germ layers - *mesoderm, endoderm* and *ectoderm* and are therefore called Mesomorph, Endomorph and Ectomorph respectively. Mesomorphs are characterized by a predominance of lean muscle, connective tissues and bone; Endomorphs are characterized by a predominant roundness & softness in the different parts of the body as a consequence of excess body fat; Ectomorphs are characterized by fragility & linearity and are therefore possess frail and weak body structures which are devoid of fat as well as lean muscle. An individual may not necessarily be a pure Somatotype and can be a combination of one or more of these Somatotypes.

These body types are not inflexible to change arising from application of stimulus in the form of exercise and diet. Not each and every one possesses a dream body shape and structure by birth. Similarly, not everyone who has the nature predisposition to a good physique is able to maintain it. The genetic code embedded into our body in the form of body type plays a significant role in determining our body shape but it is not the only parameter. It is true that an Ectomorph may ingest large number of calories as part of diet and may perform rigorous strength training routines but still may find it difficult to add an extra pound of weight. Similarly, an endomorph may perform long duration cardiovascular workouts but still may not be able to shed those extra pounds of fat stored in the body. However, genetic predisposition only indicates the difficulty to create changes; nowhere does it mention that it is impossible. Moreover, in most cases an individual is a combination of Somatotypes which makes it possible to create changes in one direction or the other depending upon the requirement. It is therefore of utmost importance to identify the body type and the goals before designing an exercise program and diet plan. Once this identification has been done, adherence to a scientifically designed weight management program will lead to achievement of the desired targets that have been set.

Components of weight management program

A healthy weight management program should be based on the four pillars of wellness – physical fitness, balanced diet & nutrition, rest & relaxation and mental attitude. A balance between all the four components is crucial for the success of a weight management program. A good fitness routine which is not accompanied by an appropriate diet will not help the individual trying to lose weight. Similarly, a person who does not have the right mental frame of mind will find it extremely difficult to adhere to certain basic restrictions that such a program may impose; as a result of which the whole program fails. A weight management program needs to be customized according the needs and goals of the individual. This customization needs to be reflected in all the components as well. In case even one of them is not in sync it can derail the whole program itself.

Balanced diet & nutrition

A good balanced and nutritious diet is paramount to the success of a weight management program. Not only should it provide the right amount of energy depending upon the goals of the program, it should also provide the necessary micronutrients in adequate quantities for long term sustainable weight loss and overall health. A balanced diet incorporates energy compounds such as carbohydrates, fats and proteins, micronutrients such as vitamins and minerals as well as fiber and water in adequate quantities. As mentioned before the quantity and proportion of the main energy compounds depends on the goal of the program while micronutrients should be available to the body as per standard guidelines such as DV (Daily Value), RDA (Recommended Dietary Allowance) and EAR (Estimated Average Requirement).

In case the goal is to lose weight then an energy deficit needs to be created in a way that energy intake is less than energy output. This may involve reducing the quantities of the energy compounds from the normal diet and vice versa in case weight gain is the goal. As part of a weight management diet plan identifying the calorie content of meals is extremely crucial. To lose one pound of fat, a deficit of 3,500 calories needs to be created. This can be done by ensuring a regular deficit of 500 calories per day throughout the week. A gradual weight loss rate of one to two pounds per week is ideal for the body since it gets time to adapt to the changed conditions. Moreover, gradual weight loss ensures that there is least amount of muscle loss that happens as part of the weight loss process. This is where the efficacy of crash diets or very low calorie diets is questioned. Apart from loss of muscle tissue they cause micronutrient deficiency extremely dangerous to overall health. Certain research studies also confirm that such diets in fact may lead to fat gain since the body experiences starvation and tends to preserve the energy dense compounds for later utilization. This is done at the expense of lean muscle tissue which is difficult to maintain in the body.

In general any meal should include around 55 to 60% energy being provided through carbohydrates, 25 to 30% energy through fats and approximately 10 to 20% through proteins. This principally ensures that while all the energy requirements are met, nourishment of the body is not compromised upon. Even in case an energy deficit is required for losing weight it created in such a way that all nutrients including fats are available to the body for essential functions that need to be performed for healthy a mind & body.

Once the energy requirements have been calculated the next step in the preparation of a balanced diet plan is identification of the meals and meal content. By identification of the meals, it is intended to finalize the meal frequency and the meal timings such that they can be incorporated in the lifestyle in an easy manner. Too many altera- tion in the existing pattern of life make the adherence to the plan that much more difficult. Therefore, a diet plan should be designed taking into consideration the individual's lifestyle and preferences. In this context the question of meal frequency becomes a pertinent one. The three meal plan has been ingrained into modern day diets since it is conveniently adopted into work life pattern. It may not necessarily be as good and efficient for overall health as well as for weight loss in comparison to a high frequency diet plan such as a 6 meal plan.

Our body requires energy at a particular rate; this rate is defined by our metabolic rate but there may be spikes in demand such as the post exercise period. Clearly, the body does not require energy at the rate at which we eat and the rate at which the energy is released in our body upon digestion of food. In such a situation the excess energy needs to be stored in the body to be utilized at a later stage. The body can do it in the form of glycogen in the liver and muscles but once these limited space stores are filled up then it converts the extra energy into fat which can be stored all over the body. Sec- ondly, whenever a heavy meal is consumed the insulin spike that occurs upon increase in glucose level in the blood, stays on for a longer period of time. In a similar manner this also results in storage of carbohydrates initially as glycogen but later on as fat. Smaller meals ensure that the body gets energy at a rate commensurate to its requirements so that it does not have to convert and store it as body fat. A high frequency 6 meal plan aids in this process of immediate utilization.

The other factor is the proportion of energy that is derived from stored energy reserves versus that derived from food that has been consume in the recent past. The body stores energy compounds like glucose in the blood, glycogen or long chain glucose molecules in the liver and muscles. And fat in the adipose tissue. Whenever the requirement for energy arises the body meets it through one of these sources. When extra carbohydrates are ingested as part of the meal the body stops utilizing the fat stored in the body, on top of this, the extra carbohydrate gets converted into fat. In a high frequency meal plan, the amount of carbohydrates consumed in any meal is limited, which prevents prolonged insulin spike from occurring. This helps in preventing conversion of carbohydrates into fat and also helps in utilizing stored fat for meeting energy requirement.

As part of weight management programs high frequency smaller meals are often suggested due to the aforementioned reasons. The other psychological advantages offered by these plans are beneficial in ensuring adherence during the initial difficult periods of change. By trimming down meal quantities and increasing frequency, cravings that lead to unplanned eating can be prevented. Since, as part of the meal itself there are many meals, the meal content is pre-planned and hence, the chances of eating something unhealthy out of the diet plan are reduce. Uncontrolled hunger pangs are also not experienced since the gap between meals is shorter. This has a dual advantage – apart from preventing binge eating it also helps in avoiding overeating during the main meals. The effect of frequent meals on metabolism has also been seen to be positive in nature. By eating frequent meals, the body is not allowed to go onto starvation mode and thereby the metabolism is maintained at a high since there it is made to experience a near constant availability of food and energy. Increased metabolism helps in burning the extra fat reserves in the body and hence helps in losing weight in a desirable manner. In summary, a high frequency smaller meal plan seems to be much more effective in reducing body fat percentage in comparison to the modern day three meal plan. This loss in fat percentage is ideal for weight loss as well as weight gain. Hence such a meal plan can be made an integral part of any weight management program.

Physical exercise as part of weight management plan

The second pillar in a healthy weight management program is regular physical exercise at the right intensity. It helps in increasing the energy output to create the deficit that is essential for weight loss to take place. In case weight gain is the goal, exercise provides stimulus forcing the body to grow to meet the additional demands placed on it. Whatever the goals may be, like a healthy weight management plan, a healthy exercise routine should include all the components – cardiovascular endurance, muscular endurance, muscular strength and flexibility.

1. Cardiovascular endurance exercises include all those exercises that involve repetitive movement of large muscle groups at a heart rate greater than resting heart rate. Exercises include running, jogging, swimming, cycling, rowing etc. The role of the cardiovascular system is to ensure efficient delivery of oxygen to different parts of the body. Performing regular cardio exercises not only improves the delivery mechanism of oxygen but also helps improve the efficiency of the vascular system and the exercising muscles to take up and utilize the oxygen delivered. Chronic adaptations as a result of cardio activities help in preventing cardiovascular and coronary artery diseases, metabolic disorders such as diabetes and metabolic syndrome and may also help in preventing certain forms of cancer.

2. Muscular endurance exercises help improve the endurance of different muscle groups in the body. Numerous activities of daily life involve repeated movements to be performed of a particular type and therefore utilize a particular muscle group. Improved muscular endurance helps in performing these movements without experiencing too much fatigue in the exercising muscle.

3. Muscular strength is the ability of a particular muscle to lift heavy loads. In daily life, the requirement to lift and carry heavy load often arises but infrequently. If the body is deconditioned to perform such a movement then there is risk of injury. Strength training exercises help in increasing lean muscle tissue in the body as well as improves the quality of

bone health by strengthening them. In such a manner it helps in performing activities of daily life.

4. Flexibility refers to pain free range of motion around a joint. This is one of the most neglected aspects of fitness and as age progresses it becomes the most important component. Flexibility training in the form of static stretches held for moderate to long durations helps in improving flexibility which then reduced the risk of injuries.

All these components of exercise are important in the context of weight management but more emphasis is directed towards exercises such as cardiovascular workouts. These exercises increase the heart rate in such a manner that the extra demands placed on the body force it to rely on stored energy reserves in the body. By careful planning of diet and intensity of workout it is possible to selectively utilize fat stored in the body for meeting the energy requirements. A balanced routine should include 40 minutes of moderate intensity aerobic activity for 3 to 4 times a week, strength training or resistance training of all the muscle groups at least twice a week and static stretching to improve flexibility should also be incorporated at least 2 to 3 times a week. Such a balanced workout leads to weight loss as well as improves overall physical fitness.

Rest & Relaxation

It is important to understand that the actual growth and development of the body does not take place while exercise is being performed. Exercise only provides the stimulus required for growth and development of tissues. The other ingredients that ensure that the purpose is fulfilled are balanced & nutritious diet and rest & relaxation. Post exercise when the body rests and is provided energy and nutrition is the time when the actual growth happens. At this stage the energy requirements should be met from within the fat stores for weight loss to take place. In case this is not done, the body will strip lean muscle tissue to meet the demands post by exercise. Also, in case enough rest is not provided to the body, the chance of overtraining leading to injury increases manifold. Adequate amount of rest and relaxation also helps in maintaining hormonal balance in the body. This is also crucial for healthy weight management.

Mental attitude

A perfectly designed diet plan or a perfectly designed exercise routine is of no use if the individual for whom it is designed is not able to adhere to it. This is where the role of a positive mental attitude comes into picture. Psychological factors play an important role in weight management than is generally imagined. In fact adherence to any plan is solely dependent on the attitude a person carries towards the lifestyle alteration that is being imposed as part of the plan. In case the weight management program is looked at as a set of limitations or restrictions that is forced, the chances of adherence in the short run as well as over a period of time diminish significantly. On the contrary an individual adopting a positive attitude looks at the program as a new positive lifestyle which is embraced with vigour and excitement.

Yoga for weight management

'Yoga' is derived from '*yuj*' in Sanskrit which means 'to unite'. Originating in ancient India, it is a unique combination of mental, physical as well as spiritual disciplines. This union that yoga refers to is the union of the individual with the universal. Yoga is believed to have originated more than 25,000 years ago and contrary to common knowledge it is not just a sequence of poses and postures for improving health and fitness. It is an ancient science that includes tools such as *pranayama* or breathing methods and techniques, meditation also called *dhyana* and finally physical postures or *asanas.*

The modern form of yoga is believed to have begun with Parliament of Religions convened in Chicago in the year 1893. In the convention *Swami Vivekanand* had a deep impact on the thinking of the audience. In subsequent tours in the United States he promoted various aspects of yoga. These talks and lectures led to yoga shedding the tag of a purely religious practice and being accepted by the western world. In the years since then health benefits emanating through regular yogic practices have been researched, documented and published all over the world. It is estimated that in the US alone more than 25 million people practice yoga on a regular basis.

The myriad benefits of yoga include physiological benefits such as improved flexibility, increased strength, better posture, weight loss, effective breathing, stronger immune system, improved bone strength and improvement in medical conditions such as migraine and insomnia; psychological benefits include stress relief, greater awareness, improved energy levels and an overall feeling of inner peace. Yoga is quite efficient in weight loss as well. It advocates a multi dimensional approach that incorporates physical, emotional and spiritual components and does not superficially work on eliminating the symptoms alone. The root cause of the problem is targeted through yoga to deal with the weight problem. It therefore involves detoxification, increasing metabolism, achieving hormonal balance, improving observation & awareness and cardiovascular endurance. Certain forms of yoga prescribe movements done at a rapid pace in a sequential manner that elevates heart rate to moderate or high levels and in such a manner mimic cardiovascular activities. This is very similar to circuit training which is a form of strength training where each muscle group is exercises one after the other without any rest. Such workout principles help in weight loss since heart rate is maintained at a moderate to high level for considerable duration. Apart from the *asanas* that are practiced, *kriyas* such as *kapalbhati* done at a vigorous intensity provides a good cardiovascular endurance workout. Different *asanas* also have different effects on the mind as well. Certain movements performed at a particular pace are known to provide calmness, while other movements help in boosting energy levels. Yoga *asanas* also improve thyroid and pituitary health and balanced secretion of hormones helps in improving metabolism to suit the body's requirements. Other benefits such as reduction in anxiety and detoxification of the body indirectly help in losing weight in a healthy manner. The psychological benefits such as improved awareness and sense of calmness help in immensely improving adherence to weight management program since they bring about a positive attitude towards the entire process.

Meditation for weight management

Meditation refers to the process of reflection and contemplation that helps in calming the mind and in this way relieves stress and anxiety. It has been commonly linked with religion and prayer across many cultures since ancient times. It is often thought of as a tool to improve concentration and as an aid to attaining peace of mind, a path to God and spirituality. Meditation is commonly done by mental exercises that include concentrated breathing, single point focussing as well as chanting. In some cultures it is performed by being completely detached from external worldly contacts while in others the person may interact with the outside world while practicing meditation.

Meditation has developed over centuries and across cultures and civilizations. There is no one form of meditation that fits all the requirements and is ideal for each and everyone practicing it. Which form suits whom depend on factors like state of mind, personality traits and external surroundings. The meditation form that should be practiced is the one in which the person feels most comfortable rather than going after something which is perceived by people in close contact to be most helpful. There is no one single source or authority or text that is referred to for meditation practices. Numerous different forms have evolved over ages each having certain distinct characteristics. A high proportion of these forms though, involve awareness of breath as the underlying platform on which meditation is practiced. Different types of meditation include the following:

1. *Mindfulness meditation* is a popular practice in the West in which awareness of the surroundings is not blocked out. The idea in this practice is to allow all the thoughts to flow into the mind without focusing on any single one of them. This form does not necessarily require quiet and peaceful surroundings and can be performed anywhere. Breathing like most meditation forms is important but is not the primary and sole element. It is a form which is suited to beginners who may find concentrating and blocking out thoughts to focus on nothingness extremely difficult.

2. *Focused meditation* involves focusing on a single thought throughout the practice session. The point of focus can be internal like an imagined object and can also be external in nature like a chant. The emphasis is not on the thought but

on the process of maintaining concentration and not losing focus.

3. *Spiritual meditation* is a form which is closely interlinked with religion and is suited to individuals who offer prayers as part of their daily rituals. The emphasis is on communication and interaction with God and union with the Universal.

4. *Trance based meditation* is an advanced form of spiritual meditation that involves reaching a state of trance by losing self control induced by usage of intoxicating substances. Since the person practicing this form of meditation may not have any memory of the experience, it has a very limited usage, if any, on daily life.

5. *Movement meditation* is a form in which the practice involves constant movement. These movements can be slow & rhythmic in nature such as swaying of the body. These gentle movements are believed to have a calming influence on the mind.

6. *Other forms of meditation* include mantra meditation, transcendental meditation, *kundalini* meditation, *Qi gong* meditation and *Zazen* meditation. Each of them originating in different ages and different parts of the world; differing in the way they are practiced and in terms of their end objectives as well.

Since it is not an exact science, the benefits of meditation cannot be directly and objectively measured. Interest in the scientific community has increased immensely as a result of observations, but studies and research has not determined conclusive proof of benefits derived from meditation. Physical benefits include elimination of stress leading to improvement in conditions such as hypertension and diabetes. The vibrations released are also known to have the added effect of diminishing the negative impact of the disease. Meditation is known to reduce the level of Cortisol and hence reduces stress levels; it also reduces the accumulation of lactic acid which is associated with anxiety. Meditation helps in breath control thereby reducing heart rate and helping the body fight against hypertension; it helps to improve immunity, provides balance to the hormonal system, improves fertility, reduces cholesterol level and helps in weight loss.

While weight loss cannot be directly achieved through meditation it has a more important role to play than any other parameter including physical exercise and diet & nutrition. Meditation does not burn fat in the body but it provides a frame of mind and attitude that is crucial for the efficient functioning of the tools that result in weight loss. Without a positive frame of mind adherence to the weight management program is practically impossible. Meditation helps in identifying the root cause of the weight problem and it does not superficially work on the symptoms of the problem. Even if an individual on a weight loss program is able to achieve weight loss, it may not be sustainable and permanent in case the root cause is not tackled. Meditation helps in improving self control and thereby increases determination that helps in adhering to the program. Moreover, the positive attitude with which the program is adopted magnifies the benefits that may be derived. From the psychological perspective of filling in voids, people have a tendency to go on binges – commonly termed as emotional eating. Meditation helps by working on elimination of desire itself helping the individual practicing it to remain unaffected by the pressures of daily home and work life. The positive attitude that is manifested helps to attain a balance in life. This balance prevents excessive emotions either positive or negative. The person thus practicing experiences an ever prevalent calmness irrespective of the external environment and the alterations that these parameters may undergo. While meditation objectively may not lead to weight loss in the conventional sense, it empowers the individual with a positive attitude – the most useful tool in attaining any weight loss goal.

Meditation also provides numerous psychological benefits. It helps ease stress & anxiety as mentioned earlier. A person becomes calm & composed and is able to visualize the external world with detachment helping in decision making process. Meditation also recharges and provides a feeling of rejuvenation which increases efficiency of all work that the person indulges in. Practicing meditation on a regular basis provides greater mental control that helps in curbing fluctuations in mood and emotion. The spiritual benefits that are derived from regular practice of meditation are manifested in the attitude of kindness and compassion towards others. Union of mind, body and soul leads to an infinite source of love. All these benefits from meditation practice helps produce a balanced personality unfazed by external events and conditions.

Conclusion

For a successful weight management program it is imperative that all these components or pillars be incorporated. When these pillars are not in sync the chances of success of these plans reduces considerably. In fact, neglecting any one of these components may compromise short term as well as long term health and wellness. On the other hand when the wavelengths of the efforts do not match it is very unlikely that the weight management goals are achieved. A positive attitude towards a weight management program that includes a well rounded physical fitness routine, a balanced diet & nutrition plan and sufficient rest & relaxation is almost a guarantee to achieving long term and sustainable weight loss.

MEDITATION

Meditation – Meaning, Types, Benefits and Impact on Weight Loss

Etymology and Meaning

Meditation is derived from the Latin verb *"meditari"* which means to think or ponder. This can further be traced back to the Hebrew language, the translation of the Hebrew Bible into Greek, led to the transformation of the root *hāgâ* into *"Melete"* (meaning *"to sigh or murmur"* and also *"to meditate")*. The Latin Bible in turned translated this root into the word on" by the Latin Bible.

A variety of words have been used to refer to "meditation" across languages and cultures e.g. the Tibetan word meditation is *"Gom"* meaning to become *"familiar with"*. This can be interpreted as familiarity to concepts positive and advantageous to our daily lives e.g. absence of fear and desire, kindness and consideration to others, tolerance, persistence etc

In modern day colloquial usage, meditation refers to the process of quiet contemplation and reflection, a process of calming the mind in order to help reduce the stress and anxiety of daily life. Sometimes it can also be linked to religion and prayer. However, to brand it in such a narrow box would be incorrect. The origin and use of mediation has spanned many centuries, across civilizations (including pre-historic), religions (Hinduism, Buddhism, Jewish, Christianity) and cultures (from India, China and Japan in the East to Europe and US in the West). In each of these the meaning and usage has taken on different nuances and meanings from an aid to peace of mind, path towards spirituality and god to a process for achievement of specific goals like concentration, compassion, detachment towards the daily life. This can also include performance of specific activities like breathing exercises, single point concentration exercises, chanting etc

The process of achieving the above can also differ from culture to religion. In some the cultures, meditation is done by being detached and cut-off from the external world and surroundings, the person having to delve within. In other forms of practice it requires the person to interact with the outside world; walking, talking, eating etc.

To summarize, there are many ways and approaches to meditation and generalizing it in a narrow definition would not be correct (similar to calling the varied art forms like writing, painting, dancing etc as the same)

History and Root

Although data suggests that some form of mediation was practiced among pre-historic civilizations (in form of chanting), written records can be traced back to 1500 BCE in Ancient India in the Vedas. In the Hindu Vedic texts it was referred to as Dhyana which comes from the Sanskrit root *"Dhyai"* meaning concentration or contemplation. Over the centuries the practice spread or developed across other countries and cultures. Although there is no clear record of the same, it is believed that the practice of meditation spread across the Eastern world around 1000 years before it spread to and gained popularity in the West.

The Buddha is known to have gained enlightenment around 500BC by sitting under the famous Banyan tree; this led to the birth of Buddhism and the Buddhist form of meditation. The text *"Pali Canon"* (a form of Buddhist scriptures) mentions meditation as a path to salvation. The silk route trade opened the doors for transmission of both Buddhism and Buddhist meditation to the other Asian countries. Over time other forms of meditation developed, Taosim in China around 5 BCE, Zen in Japan (the first meditation hall was opened in Nara, Japan in 653)

Islamic culture was also not immune to the advances of meditation, *"Dhikr"* the Islamic devotional practice of the silent recitation of the 99 names of gods can be considered a form of prayer and meditation (started around 8th / 9th century onwards). Over time Sufism (another religious practice in the Islamic word) stared to include breathing controls and repetition of words.

In western civilization, some form of meditation appears to have been mentioned around 20BCE in Greece. The writings of Philo of Alexandria hint at activities focused on attaining spirituality and aiding concentration. Around the 3rd century Plotinus had developed practices for performing meditation

Western Christian meditation developed around 6th century among monks from their practice of divine or Bible reading. Christian meditation differed from other forms in the method of its practice. As opposed to chanting / repetition of phrases, Christian meditation propagated the four formal steps of reading, pondering, praying and contemplating. In the west meditation remained in the domain of the intellectuals and saints till about the middle of the 20th century wherein it started gaining popularity among the masses as they realized the healing benefits in relieving stress, aiding relaxation and overall spiritual development.

It can be said the transmission of the knowledge about meditation came a full circle around the 1950s as a more Western and non religious form of meditation was initiated in India from the West. This then again travelled forward to the United States and Europe in the 1960s and is very similar to the more popular form of meditations as known today. This form doesn't emphasize the religious and spiritual angle of meditative techniques but focuses more on battling modern day evils like stress, and anxiety. Over time the practice of meditation has become popular enough to excite scientific curiosity also, with scientific research being performed on it in the 1970s and 1980s. However, given the various non quantifiable aspects of meditation, these studies have yet to come out with clear answers on how meditation actually works

Meditation can now truly be called a widespread and global practice with some form or the other being practices across cultures, religions and countries. In all of the above it has taken on a different mode and form, in many cases very different from the source from where it was introduced. The fact that there is no one all encompassing definition to include all the practices and desired objectives could be one of the reasons why scientists have struggled to come to any conclusive research on meditation.

Types of meditation

Just as one size of clothes cannot fit all, in a similar manner there is no one form of meditation which can be applicable everyone. Meditation has developed across many centuries, culture and countries. This has led to the development of many diverse forms of meditation with their own distinct practices and results. Which particular form is suitable to an individual can depend upon factors like personality, state of mind at the point, external surroundings etc. They key is to choose the technique with which the person is most comfortable with rather than what is considered the "in thing" at the moment.

There is no single authority / text which can be conclusively referred to for providing detailed information on the various types of meditation. However, over the years certain distinctive techniques have developed which have come to be popularly accepted as separate types. Most of them have the flow of breath as a common linking factor. While some techniques give more importance to breathing (making the inhaling and exhaling as a focal point of the technique), others make it as one of the factors to be noticed while practicing. It is not possible to provide an exhaustive list of all of the meditation techniques being practiced around the world, given their sheer number, however below we give some of the major types being practiced.

The list below lists the different types of meditation forms being practiced based on the technique, however this can also be done on the basis of the religion (e.g. meditation in Buddhism, Christianity, Hinduism, Jainism, Islam etc). Given how meditation techniques have travelled across the world, many of the above religions would have similar techniques being used.

Mindfulness Meditation

It is one of the most popular types of meditation, especially in the West. As the name suggests, it is a meditation in which one is aware of one's surroundings and does not endeavor to block out the external world and associated sounds. The idea is to let the thoughts flow through your mind but without becoming attached or focused on any particular thought. This does not necessarily require quite surroundings (though they may be useful), this can be performed in the middle of a crowded park with people all around also. The aim would be to let all the sounds just flow thorough mind in a detached manner. Some people also refer to this process as *"Vipassana"*. Breathing while important (as in most types of meditation) is not a key element here. It is one of the many thoughts and flows which go through the mind

In practice, mindfulness meditation can be useful for beginners. They are more likely to find it difficult to empty the mind and focus on nothingness and perform other more technical forms of meditation. The lack of attachment to any particular thought is what aids in relaxation of the individual.

Focused Meditation

This is the next step in taking up for advanced meditation techniques. It involves focus on a particular thought throughout the entire process. The thought can be something internal (like imagining a particular object or situation) as well as external (like a sound or a chant). The thought in itself is not important, the unwavering focus on the thought is.

Given the broad scope of the above type, there are a few offshoots to focused meditation

- Guided Visualization – This refers to focused meditation on some thought or imaginary situation. In popular usage instructors / guides asks their students to imagine their special comfort place. Some kind of external recordings can also be played to aid the imagination e.g. playing the sound of leaves rustling to facilitate thoughts of a jungle or wooded field.

- Rhythm Based Meditation - This involves focus on any bodily rhythm e.g. breathing or beating of the heart. The idea is that by giving full focus / attention to any particular rhythm, other thoughts are more likely to melt away and not disturb the mental peace. Thus a practitioner will be focusing on each inhale and exhale, controlling his / her breaths by making them deeper, slower and fuller which would prevent the mind from wandering on other external thoughts.

Mantra Meditation

In Hindu texts and philosophy it is believed that certain words provide a positive vibration when chanted or spoken out loudly. These can referred to as Mantras, for example the syllable "*Om*" (pronounced as AUM) when chanted out aloud is supposed to have many healing benefits and is used in religious ceremonies in India. Mantra meditation combines the benefits of meditations and these positive vibrations. The chanting also helps the practitioner to focus his mind and empty it of other thoughts.

In more advanced forms Mantra Meditation can be called as **Transcendental Meditation.** It emerges from the Hindu form of meditation, and while it is practiced by the chanting of a Mantra the focus is on becoming detached from all that is materialistic and transient. A practitioner in the more advanced stages of Transcendental Meditation will focus on altering the breath to actually change the state of existence with the ultimate aim of leaving the materialistic body behind (also referred to as "Samadhi" in India)

Kundalini Meditation

This is another form of meditation which has roots in Vedas in the Hindu culture. It is based on the concept that all human beings have a certain number of energy centers in their bodies with one being on top of the head also. Energy in our body is moves in an upward moving stream to this energy center on top of the head and from their into infinity (in some cases it can be considered moving into the ultimate energy source of all universe). The idea behind the meditation is to move with this rising stream of energy upwards into perpetuity. As opposed to some of the other techniques described above, this form of meditation focuses on breathing and makes it a key factor in its implementation. The meditation practitioner is supposed to concentrate on the flow of breath through each of the energy centers and finally into breathing. The focus on any one activity being performed in the body also helps to empty the mind of other unwanted thoughts.

Qi Gong Meditation

Qi Gong Meditation derives from the Taoist form of meditation where breathing is the focus of the practitioner. Similar to Kundalini meditation this form also believes in energy centers in the body and the flow of energy through them. However, in this form there are three major energy centers; forehead center, chest center and two inches below the navel. The focus is on flow of energy (via breathing) through the various organs and energy centers, but in an oval manner referred to as the *"microcosmic orbit"* (like an energy channel encircling the upper part of the body). This process of energy circulation is called as *"Qi"* or *"Chi"*. This flow of energy is supposed to improve blood circulation thereby improving the brain function by increase in secretion of some vital chemicals.

Zazen Meditation

Zazen refers to the Japanese Buddhist form of meditation. It is a more advanced form of meditation as it provides minimal guidance on how it has to be learnt and performed. It is generally done for extended time periods and only basic instructions with respect to the posture are given (sitting with a straight back). Although there is no particular focus on breathing, it can be done in combination with focus on some Buddhist scripture. Given the minimalistic approach towards instruction, it is more suited individuals in a more simple and Spartan surroundings.

Spiritual Meditation

This form of meditation is more entwined with religion as compared to others described above. It is a meditation more suited for those who anyways offer prayer on a regular basis as it is based on interaction and communication with god and the spirit world. The idea behind this technique is to empty your mind of external thoughts, become relaxed, calm and detached from the outer world and then try and feel the oneness with the spiritual forces in the world. Focusing on breathing can be a good way to start so quiet the mind, once that has been achieved the mind is more free to explore the link between the conscious and sub conscious world.

Trance Based Meditation

This can be considered a more advance form of Spiritual Meditation. In some spheres this is not considered a proper form of meditation as there is a lack of self control and can at times involves the usage of intoxicants or hypnotism to produce the trance like state. This form of mediation is characterized by an absence of control, rational thinking and the feeling of no longer being part of the body. If this effect has been produced by external stimulus (hypnotism or intoxicants) then memory of experiencing this mediation can be limited for the practitioner. This can be a negating factor at times because without knowledge of the control gained over the mind, the use in daily life can be limited. Apart from intoxicants and hypnotism music and even rapid breathing can be used to induce this state.

Movement Meditation

As the name suggests, unlike all of the above forms of meditation, under this technique the practitioner has to move to meditate. There are no fixed movements to perform this; they can be slow and rhythmic like the gentle swaying of the body, hands, head, etc, the gentle movements helping to calm the mind. They can also be fast and intense movements to breakthrough some stubborn thoughts and molds in our thoughts and body, post which a more calming state can be achieved. The practice of *"Osho"*, which has gained a lot of popularity over the last few years draws heavily from this form of meditation.

While the above forms and techniques outline some of the more popular forms of meditation being practiced today, it is virtually impossible to compile and exhaustive list given the many offshoots of each of the above techniques which exist and are being created even as we speak. Different cultures adopt a particular kind of technique and then adapt it to their own surroundings to create a new form of meditation.

Benefits of Meditation

Meditation is not an exact science. While over the past many years there has been an increase in scientific interest in meditation and its many benefits, there have been no conclusive or authoritative results on what meditation is, how it works and what are its benefits. However, having said that, there are many benefits (and even miracles) which have been attributed to meditation over the centuries. These range from the physical to the metaphysical. Broadly speaking, the benefits of meditation can be broken down into three broad categories Physical or Health Related, Mental or Psychological and Spiritual

Physical or Health related benefits

In modern day lifestyles stress is the cause of many of our health problems, from heart diseases to diabetes to hypertension. While meditation is not a medicine which can scientifically cure the disease itself, it helps to attack these problems at the root to prevent their occurrence and minimize the negative impact if the person is already suffering from them. Meditation can provide a two-fold benefit here. Meditative techniques provide a calming effect and help reduce stress thereby preventing the onset of the diseases and the positive energy / vibrations released help reduce the negative impact of the diseases. Meditation helps reduce the production of Cortisol (hormone associated with stress levels). Studies have shown that regular meditation helps to increase the strength of alpha waves being produced in the body, these alpha waves are associated with a peaceful and quiet state of the mind (similar to sleep). This relaxed state further inhibits the production of lactic acid in the blood associated with high anxiety levels.

Given below are some of the many health related benefits of meditation which people have experienced over the years (as stated above, these are not medically or scientifically proven benefits, but those which many people have experienced as they practiced meditation).

1. Breadth control in meditation helps to slow the body down, its heart rate and oxygen utilization rate. This helps in fighting against hypertension, blood pressure, anxiety attacks

2. Meditation is also known to strengthen the immune system which helps in fortifying the body against germs and viruses and also aids in healing (be it from the common cold to post-op recovery)

3. Meditation is known to help balance the hormonal system which can help women before and during the menstruation cycle. Hormonal balance can also help both men and women in emotional control in their daily lives.

4. Meditation can help control cholesterol levels which can help in fighting heart diseases and diabetes.

5. Meditation is also known to help control weight problems and in aiding weight loss (more details on this later).

6. Meditation overall improves the health and well-being of an individual which makes them more energetic and positive in their approach.

7. Meditation is also known to increase sperm and ovulation count in men and women, which in turn helps battle infertility. This also could be attributed to the reduction of stress and tension which is known to have a negative impact on sperm and ovulation count.

8. Meditation improves stress levels which help control anger and temper and their harmful side-effects on the human body.

9. Recent scientific studies have concluded that meditation can also transform the brain and alter brain activity. Scientific experiments conducted have shown that there was a change in the grey matter of people who were doing regular meditation. There was an increase noticed in parts of the brain responsible for memory, learning and emotional quotient and decrease in those associated with anxiety and stress

Mental or Psychological Benefits

Meditation provides a number of psychological benefits also. As mentioned above, meditation helps in the production of alpha waves which help ease anxiety and stress. Meditation slows down the frantic pace of brain activity brought out by our over-crowded lives. This does not mean that the person becomes less intelligent or capable, as the level of awareness actually improves. It just means that the person becomes calm and composed, able to view the external world in a more detached manner which helps in decision making. People who practice meditation regularly feel rejuvenated and recharged post meditation, increasing their efficiency in whatever work they choose to do. This serene and tranquil state leads to a host of benefits, some of which have been outlined below.

1. One of the most important benefits of practicing meditation is mental control. Regular practice enables the practitioner to prevent the minds from moving from thought to thought and to focus it on a particular subject. This improves the mental sharpness, capability and concentration of a person making him / her much more efficient in any work they perform

2. Mental control also leads to control over moods and emotions. Regular practice can help control moods swings, extreme displays of negative emotions such as anger, jealousy, hate etc.

3. Increase in control not only makes a person more likable but also helps improve self confidence and self esteem.

4. Regular practice also helps a person to overcome their phobias and fears. People start seeing the phobias for what they are, imaginary situations / events / people etc which have been blown out of proportion by an overstressed and overworked mind.

5. A meditative person becomes a better listener. He / she is able to better understand what others are saying, exhibit self control in times of extreme emotional outbursts by the other, and is overall able to behave in much more healthier and mature manner. All of these help the person to form and sustain better and longer lasting relationships both in their professional and personal set up.

6. Meditation helps to calm the mind. A stressed person's brain is overloaded with multitude of thoughts, each pushing and shoving to get mind space. More likely than not such a person is likely to suffer from insomnia as some thought or the other is keeping him / her awake. Meditation helps to sort out all of these thoughts and clear the mind, leading

to a healthy sleep. Such people do not have to sleep long hours also as the hours they have slept have been refreshing enough for the mind.

7. Focus and concentration make a person sharper, more alert and better able to solve react in a sudden problem situation. This improves the problem solving skills of the person.

8. A healthy mind and body leading to a happy and fulfilling life obviate the need of external stimulus or intoxicants (hypnosis, drugs, smoking, liquor etc) to help produce a happy and satisfied state. This helps to combat drug and other forms of substance abuse.

9. Meditation is also known to foster the creative aspects of the brain

10. All of the above benefits help produce a well rounded and balanced personality, able to handle a variety of situations with ease.

Spiritual Benefits

One of the biggest advantages of meditation is the spiritual aspects. Practitioners, especially regular practitioners are able to rise above their daily lives and routine and observe things from a more broader and holistic manner. It is said that human beings use just a fraction of their brains in their daily lives. Meditation helps us to harness the energy in the remaining part and develop the subconscious self. This can bring about immense change in the personality of the individual, with the chores of the daily life not seeming arduous any more, and the person becoming more involved in questions like the purpose of life itself. Some of the spiritual benefits and changes which can be observed by practicing meditation are

1. Increase in kindness and consideration towards others – One of the basic benefits of meditation is reduction in hostility towards the external environment. Meditation helps bring a peace of mind which improves acceptance of and tolerance towards others. This forms the building block, from this stems the knowledge that all of us are on the same path towards self realization, this unity of pur-

pose in turn increases kindness and consideration towards others

2. Synchronization between the body (physical), mind (ego) and soul (spirit) – One of the biggest causes of conflict in our lives is the disagreement between the mind, body and soul. With a clash in their purposes the self gets torn between various actions (with the body and mind living more in the physical world and the soul concerned with the cosmic). Meditation reduces our dependence and desire for the physical world and helps bridge this gap.

3. Reduced emphasis on the ego- Most people are very caught up in their image of themselves. At times this desire to "be someone" becomes an obsessive force which prevents us from enjoying our lives. Meditation helps us to realize that the physical self is a tiny part in the universe and in our wider calling providing much needed humility to our lives.

4. Acceptance, of external as well as internal events – There are many teachers who preach that the external world is an ephemeral part of our lives and there is a wider and deeper meaning to our lives. However, at times, events in this transient life can cause us much hurt and pain. These emotions stem from our non-acceptance of the events happening in our lives, a master is rarely perturbed by events around him / her. Meditation helps us gain this perspective and increases our acceptance.

5. Infinite capacity for love – Meditation provides us with a wider understanding of the world around us. It makes us realize that each individual / soul is on the path of self discovery and their acts and deeds are just an unconscious way of reaching the path. This not only makes us more forgiving towards them but the unity of our goal increases our love towards them. Meditation also makes us realize that love can answer many more questions and open many more doors than hate. We start to understand how much more true and complete joy is there in spreading love than jealousy and hatred.

6. Communion with god – All of the above take us step by step closer toward the creator. We start to realize in believe in a loving and compassionate god who is always there to help us in times of need. Regular meditation can hasten our spiritual union with god

7. Helps attain "Nirvana" or enlightenment – This is the final stage of masters and teachers. When there is realization of our true purpose on earth, when the daily lives and responsibilities are left behind for a higher calling. Meditation helps answer the question "Who am I and why am I here".

To summarize, there are multitude benefits of meditation, ranging from the physical to the spiritual. Depending upon the level of practice and expertise of the practitioner, he / she is able to move higher up the ladder and avail of more advantages. Different types of meditation listed above have different advantages and can be chosen accordingly as per the goal of the practitioner.

Meditation and Weight Loss

People always associate weight loss with proper eating and regular exercise, sitting quietly (even motionless) in place generally doesn't fall into the category of "things to do for weight loss". While meditation is less effective in actually burning the fat like a workout does, it is extremely important in creating the right kind of (internal) atmosphere needed for losing the weight. Exercise in itself can be pointless if we continue to have a negative approach or are irregular in our efforts. Below are some of the reasons why mediation is an invaluable tool to help is in shedding those extra pounds.

1. Helps identify the root of our weight problem – Without identifying the source of the weight issues, exercise and diet can often be in vain. Even if the individual is able to lose weight, it is unlikely to be permanent until the root cause has also been addressed. For example many people tend to binge eat when angry, stressed, unhappy etc. Thus no matter how hard they try, weight loss techniques are unlikely to be successful or permanent until they are able to bring some peace

and calm in their life or break the vicious circle between extreme emotions, eating and weight gain.

2. Increased determination and self control – Weight loss is not just about the physical activity or restriction of calorie intake, there are many more factors at work to get that perfect figure or body. A person can have the best of intentions about losing weight, but without the mental control and determination to put these into practice, chances of success are slim. Just knowing that they have to exercise regularly and reduce high calorie food is not useful; it is the doing which is going to help achieve the results. Meditation can help bring this focus and determination. One of the many benefits of meditation is self control, focus and single-mindedness of purpose, which help in weight loss.

3. Reduces comfort eating – One of the most common reasons for gaining weight are stress and anxiety eating. Many people who find a void in their lives tend to fill it with food. This is frequently referred to as emotional eating and is not done out of a physical desire for food but emotional desire of fulfillment. Meditation helps a person focus inwards and reduces the need for external praise and acceptance. When the sense of fulfillment is coming from within, external stimulus in the form of food is no longer required. Recent studies have indicated that even extreme positive emotions can cause excessive eating as the body is not able to distinguish between extreme positive and negative stimulus. Meditation helps to bring a more balanced approach to life and thinking which negates the impact of both extreme positive and negative reactions

4. Reduction in desire – A corollary of the above benefit is the decrease in desire itself. As has been stated above in the "Benefits of Meditation" sector, a regular practitioner rises above the chores and pressures of daily lives. He / she realizes that our physical existence is just a means to achieve a higher goal. This leads to a reduction in dependence and desire on external stimuli. Masters and ascetics have been

known to survive little or no food for extended periods of time. While this is an extreme example of highly developed individuals, regular practitioners are also able to achieve a reasonable reduction in desire in their daily lives, which in turn can help in weight loss.

5. Positive thoughts/ visualization help achieve the goal – Many studies have shown that positive thinking is an essential tool in achieving any goal (whether it be a desired job, promotion or weight loss). It has been shown that a person's thoughts can be a strong force in creating his / her reality. Thus a person is imagining himself /herself to be overweight and fat, is likely to negate the positive effects of regular exercise and healthy eating. Meditation helps to control the minds and push out any negative thoughts and fears, to be replace with positive, healthy and more conducive thoughts

6. Provides a balanced approach to thinking, thereby limiting both binge eating and starvation – Meditation helps to reduce excessive emotions. A regular practitioner is less likely to be affected by both extreme positive or negative news. Studies have shown that habitual eating can at times be caused by strong emotions, thus limiting their impact on the self is likely to help in weight loss. Meditation also provides a measure of balanced thinking in life; regular practitioners are less likely to be impatient for immediate results as they will realize that all things happen at their own time and pace. This is apt to reduce the need for severe crash diets followed by equally strong binge eating sessions as the body starts to crave food.

7. Helps control hormones associated with weight gain – Apart from the mental benefits of meditation on weight gain, it also helps by controlling the secretion of negative hormones. Studies have shown that Cortisol (hormone associated with increased stress levels) also inhibits the body's ability to fight fat deposits. Meditation helps to reduce the production Cortisol in our body which in turn helps with weight loss.

8. Helps improve "Mindfulness" –Meditation helps a person become more mindful or aware of what they are doing. Thus in the case of compulsive eaters, meditation can make them aware of why they are eating, what they are eating, how much, are they actually taking pleasure in the eating or is it just a mechanical activity being performed. This helps in reducing "habit" part of eating and replaces it with "need", thereby helping in weight loss.

There have been studies done in which groups of people have been taught meditation and given lessons on mindful eating alongside with regular meditation. Results have shown that people who were able to successfully learn mindful eating and meditation had a drop in their Cortisol levels and experienced more weight loss than the others. The weight loss can be attributed to the reduced Cortisol levels and also sensory changes in the brain associated with hunger and desire.

The purpose of the above points is not to claim that weight loss can be achieved by performing meditation alone (although such cases have also been there). The purpose is to illustrate that meditation is an extremely useful tool in the entire process of weight loss. It can speed up and improve the effectiveness of the other weight loss means being used (e.g. exercise and calorie control). By helping a person visualize himself/ herself in a more positive manner, meditation is able to harness the energy of the subconscious mind to aid in weight loss.

Body goals diary

_____

_____

_____

_____

_____

_____

_____

_____

_____

_____

_____

_____

_____

_____

Body goals diary

_____

_____

_____

_____

_____

_____

_____

_____

_____

_____

_____

_____

Body goals diary

_____

_____

_____

_____

_____

_____

_____

_____

_____

_____

_____

_____

_____

_____

Body goals diary

_____

_____

_____

_____

_____

_____

_____

_____

_____

_____

_____

_____

_____

_____

Body goals diary

_____

_____

_____

_____

_____

_____

_____

_____

_____

_____

_____

_____

_____

_____

Body goals diary

_____

_____

_____

_____

_____

_____

_____

_____

_____

_____

_____

_____

_____

Body goals diary

_____

_____

_____

_____

_____

_____

_____

_____

_____

_____

_____

_____

_____

_____

_____

Body goals diary

_____

_____

_____

_____

_____

_____

_____

_____

_____

_____

_____

_____

Body goals diary

Body goals diary

_____

_____

_____

_____

_____

_____

_____

_____

_____

_____

_____

_____

_____

Body goals diary

_____

_____

_____

_____

_____

_____

_____

_____

_____

_____

_____

_____

_____

_____

Body goals diary

_____

_____

_____

_____

_____

_____

_____

_____

_____

_____

_____

_____

_____

Body goals diary

_____

_____

_____

_____

_____

_____

_____

_____

_____

_____

_____

_____

_____

_____

Body goals diary

_____

_____

_____

_____

_____

_____

_____

_____

_____

_____

_____

_____

_____

Body goals diary

_____

_____

_____

_____

_____

_____

_____

_____

_____

_____

_____

_____

_____

_____

_____

Body goals diary

_____

_____

_____

_____

_____

_____

_____

_____

_____

_____

_____

_____

_____

Body goals diary

_____

_____

_____

_____

_____

_____

_____

_____

_____

_____

_____

_____

_____

_____

Body goals diary

_____

_____

_____

_____

_____

_____

_____

_____

_____

_____

_____

_____

Body goals diary

_____

_____

_____

_____

_____

_____

_____

_____

_____

_____

_____

_____

_____

_____

_____

Body goals diary

_____

_____

_____

_____

_____

_____

_____

_____

_____

_____

_____

_____

About the author

C. T. Pam is not a physician, rather she is a regular person who has explored many avenues of eating healthy and finding a healthy lifestyle balance. After a car accident in 2010 left her unable to continue running, she found a work-life balance that has helped her maintain a healthy lifestyle. C. T. Pam has a B.A. in Political Science and Studio Art, an MBA with a entrepreneurship concentration and is currently pursuing a doctoral degree with a research focus in Entrepreneurship.

Book description

This book includes sound advice and facts regarding

- Introduction to weight management
- Choosing meal portions

While this book doesn't intend to tell the reader the best way to lead a healthy lifestyle, the author advises the reader to take away items that he or she can realistically achieve. You won't lose 50 pounds overnight, and you will have an opportunity to explore options that might benefit your physical, emotional and lifestyle needs. This book includes pages for the reader to record their goals and progress.

Volume 4 is an excerpt from Adopting a healthy lifestyle (1-884711-34-0)

Also available from Innovative Publishers

Introduction to the Paleo diet. (978-1884711466)

Introduction to the Paleo diet + 200 recipes (1884711820)

Love is... (978-1884711138)

Extreme Betrayal (978-1884711084)

Beware the Bumble Bee (978-1884711091)

Doing business with the U. S. government (978-1884711107)

Visit http://innovative-publishers.com for ordering information

Find us online @

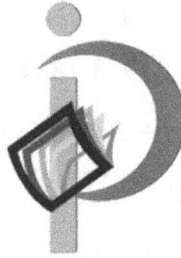

Innovative Publishers

 InnovaPub

 www.innovative-publishers.com

 pub@innovative-publishers.com

 http://innovativepublishers.blogspot.com/

 http://www.facebook.com/InnovativePublishers

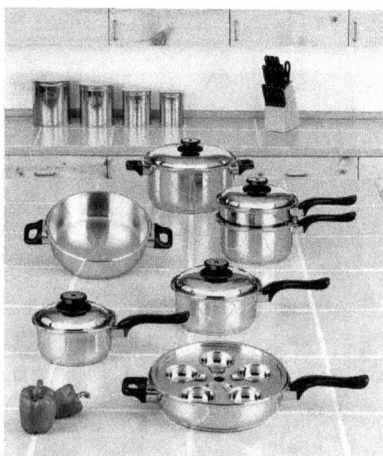

World's Finest™ 7-Ply Steam Control™ 17pc T304 Stainless Steel Cookware Set

Each piece is constructed of extra-heavy stainless steel and guaranteed to last a lifetime. Steam control valves make "waterless" cooking easy and the 7-ply construction spreads heat quickly and evenly, allowing one stack to cook. Cookware is also equipped with superbly styled phenolic handles resistant to heat, cold and detergents. Comes with a limited lifetime warranty. White box.

Suggested Retail Price : $2195.00

Item Number : GGKT17ULTRA

Set Contents

- 1.7Qt Covered Saucepan
- 2.5Qt Covered Saucepan
- 3.2Qt Covered Saucepan
- 7.5Qt Covered Roaster
- 11-3/8" Skillet, Double Boiler Unit With Capsule Bottom That You Can Also Use As An Extra 3Qt Saucepan
- 5 Egg Cups
- 5 Hole Utility Rack And High Dome Cover With Capsule Bottom So You Can Use As A Frypan
- Cover Fits Skillet Or Roaster

Features

- Extra-Heavy Stainless Steel Construction
- Heat-Resistant Phenolic Handles
- 7-Ply Construction

Limited Lifetime Warranty

» Estimated Case Weight : 36.55 Lbs.

61   Advertisement

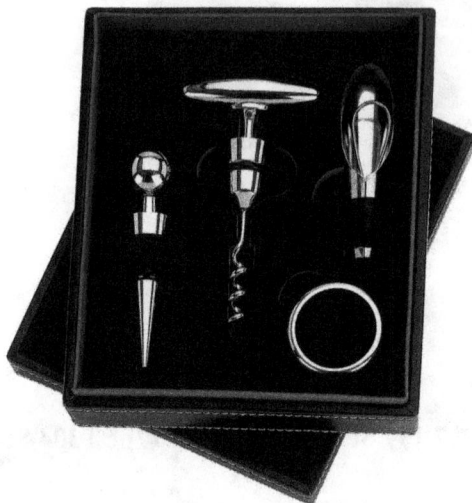

Wyndham House™ 4pc Wine Set in Storage Case

Wyndham House™ wine sets are a great compliment to any home bar, and are sure to add to the ease and elegance of wine presentations. Includes stainless steel wine spout, stainless steel wine ring, zinc alloy screw opener, and zinc alloy wine stopper. All enclosed in a 6-3/8" x 5-5/8" x 2-1/4" faux leather case.

Suggested Retail Price : $32.95

Next Ship Date : 01/05/2013

Item Number : GGKTWINE4

Features

- Stainless Steel Wine Spout
- Stainless Steel Wine Ring
- Zinc Alloy Screw Opener
- Zinc Alloy Wine Stopper
- 6-3/8" X 5-5/8" X 2-1/4" Faux Leather Case

Shipping Details

» Estimated Piece Weight : 1.10 Lbs.

62

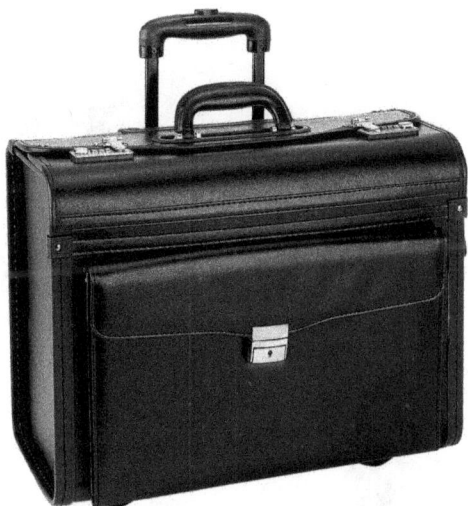

Embassy™ Sample/Pilot Case with Aluminum Trolley

Features PVC matte black exterior, rolling wheels, gunmetal combination locks, carrying handle, 2 exterior pockets, interior dividers, interior pockets, and pen holders. Measures 19" x 14" x 9".

Suggested Retail Price : $233.95

Number : BCPILOT3

Features

- Pvc Matte Black Exterior
- Rolling Wheels
- Gunmetal Combination Locks
- Carrying Handle
- 2 Exterior Side Pockets
- Interior Dividers & Pockets
- Pen Holders
- Measures 18" X 13" X 8"

Shipping Details

» Estimated Piece Weight : 8.70 Lbs.

To order products, go to the Innovative Publishers website and click Client specials. Clients receive up to 70% off the suggested retail price.